DANIEL MCKENZIE

CW00866904

ACKNOWLEDGMENTS

I would like to take the time to acknowledge the plethora of resource that I found on the web in relation to Ketogenesis, for and against alike; as the opinions and data I found were instrumental in helping me to form my own views. I think it would be futile to try to name every person or website I researched, so I won't, however I am grateful.

This book is in part based on my own weight loss results, as well as those of Alison Hope, Carol Ellis-Martin and Harpreet Harry Singh, who I'd like to thank for putting your faith in these writings, and having the gumption to give the diet a go, given what you'd been taught and believed about nutrition. Your help tested what I had researched, and I'm glad that like me you are all reaping the rewards of ketogenesis and the Ketogenic diet

Preface

So do you want to lose weight? Well, if the answer is yes, go ahead and buy this book, but! And yes there is a but. If you're serious about losing weight, and when I say weight, I specifically mean fat, I urge you, once bought, please, please, please, follow what I've laid out throughout the book, as I believe that you'll attain great fat reduction results by the end of your first week, and huge weight loss results over a three month period.

Before we start, I must first tell you that I am no physician, scientist, nutritionist or anything like that. (Though after what I have researched, I am now seriously thinking about taking a course.) Rather, I am just a guy who has struggled with weight issues for most of my adult life, and after stumbling on some inspiring information coupled with some painstaking research and fantastic weight loss results, I feel that I must pass on what I've learned about weight loss to people who are in a similar situation.

To most of you this book will seem radical, and will go against everything that you've been taught and believe about nutrition, however, it's not rocket science, indeed, here I have tried to lay out the science behind the diet simply, this is stuff that I think you'll be able to research yourself if you want to and will hopefully understand.

But first a little more about me: My name is Daniel McKenzie, and as I alluded to earlier I've struggled to keep my weight down for as long as I can remember. I think I was

Do You Want to Lose Weight?

By Daniel McKenzie

ISBN-13: 978-1505339598
ISBN-10: 1505339596

thin once. I must have been five years old or something like that, but as soon as I reached adolescence I begain to pile on the pounds.

Throughout the years I think I must have tried every conceivable diet, Atkins, Cabbage soup, the flat belly diets, Low fat, Low carb, Low protein diets, The Mediterranean diet, Slim fast, Weight Watchers, The grapefruit diet, The five two fasting diet and a plethora of others. To be quite honest, some were better than others; and while some were healthy, quite a lot were certainly not. There were those where I lost pounds, only to pile the weight and more back on again while still on the diet, my body being forced into starvation mode, my metabolism slowing and my fat cells filling almost uncontrollably.

In addition to the diets, I spent hundreds of pounds on Gym memberships, hitting the treadmill, weight room and exercise bike, sweating buckets, only to get swollen joints, aching muscles and seeing no real benefits. So in the end I did what most people who struggle with weight issues do. I gave up.

Is that what we really do? I suppose not. I did try to live healthily, you know, doing what I was told to do by my physician and the media. I cut my saturated fat intake, only ate so many eggs per week, cut down on the processed meat and sugars; you know the spiel? All that stuff that healthy looking physicians, scientist and the media executives bombard us with on a daily basis. But my weight still rose, and rose, to a point to where I got seriously ill.

I ended up in hospital as a 20 stone (280 pounds) shadow of

a residual self image. Seeing images now of what I was like back then shows me how much I had let myself go, however in my mind's eye I was nowhere near as fat as I really was, but who was I kidding? Suffice it to say, I almost died; I faced multiple organ failure and spent a couple of weeks in hospital in an intensive care unit. Anyway, it turns out, my liver and pancreas seem to have had enough of the rich living and rebelled and it seemed like I had one choice. That was to lose weight.

That was five years ago, and since then I've been on one diet or other; you know back into the same old routine. As before, my weight yo-yoed as I skipped from diet to diet; I became a gym rat once more, sore muscles and aching joints to look forward to and taking supplements to build muscle to rid me of that dreaded fat.

I must say, I did obtain good results and up until a six months ago I had shed 5 stones (70 pounds), however, from what I was told, again from my physician, I had at least 1.5 stones (21 pounds) to lose before I left the lower end of the obese zone. Unfortunately for me I had been at that weight for eighteen months, yo-yoing up and down four or five pounds every few weeks, and no matter what I tried, I just could not shift the weight.

I'd played around with my diet and started with low fat, low carb and high protein, then low fat, high carb and moderate protein, then low fat, moderate carb and moderate protein, then restricted this and upped that. I tell you, I got so sick of the permutations and the lack of weight loss, plus beating myself up in the gym, that I nearly gave up once more. In the end I just tried to eat sensibly and had a few less gym days. I took consolation in telling myself that I had come a long way, I mean 5 stones (70 pounds) was not to be sniffed at? But deep down I needed to lose the rest.

I thought about cancelling my gym membership as up until that point I had done a little research into diet and had learned that no amount of gym work would help if ones diet was bad, but what could I do? I had reached the end.

Six months ago whilst scouring the web for a close friend, in search for ways of slowing down the onset of dementia, I came across several articles which, promoted the use of coconut oil to slow it down. OK, this was different I thought. A few days later I read an article in one of the national newspapers, then a couple of days after that I heard a news report raving about the use of coconut oil and how it was being used on Alzheimer's patients, with varying degrees of success in slowing down the onset of memory loss.

But with the taking of coconut oil would the patients not put on weight, get fat and have heart attacks? What would the physicians do to prevent this from happening? I mean, as far back as I could remember we were taught about the dangers of the consumption of saturated fats. They clog up the arteries don't they?

After a bit more research I found something astonishing. I found that the consumption of fat had been used for thousands of years for ailments such as memory loss, epilepsy, cancer therapy and a host of others, even weight loss. Weight loss eh... This had just become interesting.

I decided to dig deeper and explored how fat could aid in weight loss. I found lots of passionate but conflicting points of view, studies that had been conducted dating back to the nineteenth century, long forgotten ailment remedies using fat which had given way to modern medicine. It was intriguing, yet a nightmare as I had no idea who I should believe. I mean my research showed me that we the public should have been questioning the mainstream, as for years we were advised to consume things that were no good for us, food stuffs that could kill us. The consumption of Trans Fats being a classic example. So I began to question why 99% of physicians believe that we, the masses should steer clear of saturated fats and cholesterol forming foods and eat their so called balanced diet.

Anyway, it wasn't long before I found several websites that talked about research that took place in the USA back in the fifties when a serious spike in the heart attack rate (cardiovascular disease) occurred. The findings of the research concluded that saturated fat was the cause, and it wasn't long before we saw low fat hydrogenated unsaturated margarine sold in our shops. And, right now even though most people eat low fat this, and low fat that, we seem to be in the midst of an obesity epidemic; well in the western world, with cardiovascular disease the biggest killer and It's on the increase, so what are we doing wrong? We are sixty years on and things have got worse and we are getting fatter.

With this in mind, I began to doubt what I had been taught about the consumption of fat throughout my life, or was this doubt down to me not being able to attain my ideal weight?

Perhaps a little of both played a part, but with this doubt in mind, I searched for more evidence or more findings that promoted that fat consumption could indeed lead to weight loss.

I didn't have to look far, as on the web there are many articles, including YouTube testimonies that promote the consumption of fat to actually target and burn fat from one's body. It was astounding; the way these individuals looked; lean, healthy and claiming that their daily fat consumption was up to 80% of their dietary intake but no less than 70%.

These people claimed that they ate all those bad things that physicians would have a heart attack about if they knew you were eating them. Cheese, double cream, butter, whole eggs, coconut oil, bacon and a long list of those crazy things that were suppose to clog the arteries.

How?

I'll tell you about my diet and how I safely lost 1.5 stones (21 pounds) in two and a half months; just continue reading.

Chapter 1: Why Did I Get Fat In The First Place - The Science Behind The Diet

As I said earlier, I want to keep this as simple as possible, as this book is meant to concentrate on the diet rather than the science. So no fancy food images, I won't go into minute detail and will be rather general. However, I do say before embarking on this, there is no reason why you shouldn't do some research yourself.

Anyway, I think it's important that understanding how and why we get fat is a good place to start, so I want you to keep the following thought in the forefront of your mind. Insulin is produced by your body to lower blood sugar levels. However, it is the only hormone in the body that can transport fat that has been derived from carbohydrates ,to your fat cells.

How this works.

When you eat carbohydrates, and I mean anything from fruit and green vegetables, to bread, rice and pasta, to sugar, cookies and cakes, all of these are broken down in to smaller particles and then eventually into glucose which then hits your blood stream ready to be used. When your body recognises that there is glucose present in your blood it signals your pancreas to produce insulin.

Remember, insulin is produced to lower blood sugar levels in our bodies, so it starts to do its' work and transports a glucose derived energy called glycogen to your liver, muscles, brain etc, ready to be used when needed. When these parts of your body have had enough, the insulin continues to lower your blood sugar and transport surplus energy to your fat cells where it is stored as free fatty acid, ready to be used by your body as a secondary energy source. The insulin will begin to lower but may be present in your blood for a few hours yet.

So, suppose I'd just eaten a fresh jam and cream filled doughnut, my insulin levels would spike as my body rushes to reduce my blood sugar level. My liver, muscles, brain etc will fill with energy and my fat cells will take up any surplus. This would happen fairly quickly, over say a couple of hours, thus leaving my blood sugar level low, and if my blood sugar level is low, I am naturally going to feel hungry, so I have some pasta and meatballs. Once again my blood sugar level spikes and even though the insulin from my first meal has not depleted, more insulin is pumped into my blood. As my muscles are already full, there is only one place the insulin will place the resulting energy. Yes, into my fat cells. And the cycle continues.

Is insulin the villain? I mean it's the only hormone that will allow our fat cells to fill. But we need insulin to live, without it my blood would be treacle and my heart wouldn't be able to pump it. A quandary.

Let me take you back to that research that took place back in the 1950s which, concluded that saturated fats were the cause of the then spike in heart attacks. Well in 1950s Americas for the first time had more disposable cash, and spent more time eating out. So rather than eating wholesome home cooked meals, they spent time in fast food restaurants etc. For the first time, they were consuming vast amounts of carbohydrates in the form of sugars, in everything from fizzy sodas, milkshakes, cereals, breads, tinned meats and vegetables etc. At that time sugars such as High Fructose Corn syrup found its way into the food chain and subsequently into nearly all food types, which meant that people were unwittingly consuming vast amounts of carbohydrates.

And Remember that:

Carbohydrate Consumption = Insulin Production

Insulin Production = Filling Fat Cells and Low Blood Sugar

Low Blood Sugar = Hunger

Hunger = Carbohydrate Consumption

So it's not surprising then, that there was a spike in the heart attack rate and its even less surprising that after sixty years of the public consuming low fat foods there is still an obesity epidemic, and cardiovascular disease is at its highest rate. You see fat is not the problem, sugar is.

Well, I suppose fat could be the problem just like we've been told: Listen, I know that I've just contradicted myself, but there is something else that you must know before embarking on this diet, which is, fat consumption can be an issue depending on what you consume it with.

Say you've just consumed that large bowl of pasta which breaks down into glucose and effects your body just as I've explained. But just think what your fat cells would look like if the pasta you consumed contained fat, say in the form of meatballs and pasta sauce. The carbohydrates in the pasta breaks down into glucose which spikes your insulin, which in turn transports excess glucose to your fat cells in the form of fatty acids. As well as this happening the fat from the meatballs and pasta sauce also fill your fat cells. A double whammy!

So this is what happens pretty much every time you eat a mixture of carbohydrate and fat, so the next time you crave that jam and cream filled doughnut, spare a thought for your fat cells.

Saying all that, perhaps the solution is more simple; perhaps we just consume more calories than we expend, and in many cases this has got to be true. But as I said earlier, and believe me, I worked hard in the gym throughout the years and had been calorie counting for, I don't know, more time than I can remember. So for me the calories in verses calories out scenario, just doesn't completely stack up.

And as I'm telling it like it is; there is an array of research out there supporting my stance and to be fair a lot more that doesn't. But if you're like me and have been dieting forever, you'll know that half of the time you're hungry, and you still can't shift the weight. For me, one more diet was not going to hurt, was it?

Chapter 2: How The Diet Works and Getting Started

To be clear, this is not a crash diet, where you do it for a few months to lose the pounds, just to pile the weight all back on again, I think we've all been down that road, rather it's a lifestyle change that you will adopt. Therefore, you won't be on a diet as such, you'll have just changed your diet, or modified what you consume.

So to much fanfare: My diet is the "Ketogenic" Diet, some of you will have heard of it, but most of you will have not. It's essentially a high-fat, sufficient protein, low-carbohydrate diet that in medicine is used primarily to treat epilepsy in children. A spin off of the use of the diet is that the body is forced to burn fats rather than carbohydrates. That's right, you read it correctly. The body is forced to burn fat.

And yes another low carb diet, one of which, I hasten to add, I'd not tried during my lifelong struggle with weight issues. At first just the thought of consuming high amounts of fat turned me off as I was already fat and had no need of more. But after doing the research: What I've just explained in relation to fat, I believed the science to be sound, it just made sense.

I decided that I had nothing to lose if I tried this diet, I mean, I'd tried many others with varying successes and spectacular failures. I would try this for a month just to see what would happen, so you can imagine how I felt when I lost six pounds in the first week.

Yes I know, some people may think, six pounds in one week was and is a bit excessive but at least four pound of this weight was derived from water weight loss. But a loss none the less.

On the diet you'll be consuming fewer carbohydrates so your body instead of looking for its' preferred primary source of energy which is derived from carbohydrates, will become fat adapted and automatically look to burn fat as its primary source. It is important to note that your brain cannot use fat as an energy source, so whilst on the diet your brain will get your liver to produce a substance called Ketone Bodies, which is something the brain can use as energy. At this stage your body is said to be in a state of Ketosis, hence the name of the diet, Ketogenic.

As I said, you'll be consuming fewer carbohydrates, but just how much less? Well there are varying schools of thought in this regard. Some practitioners say go as low as 15 grams per day, and others say as much as 100 grams. You will note that 100 grams of carbohydrates is pretty low compared to 250 grams for women and 300 grams for men, which are the approximate daily recommended levels of carbohydrate consumption for adults. This means bread, pasta, rice, potatoes, sugars in its' varying forms, and many fruits will go from your diet. Remember these are the things that can raise your insulin levels and that's what has to be avoided.

My Diet:

The following shows my macronutrient consumption before I embarked on the Ketogenic diet.

Carbohydrates 120 grams = 480 calories

Protein 100 grams = 400 calories

Fat 70 grams = 630 calories

Total calories = 1510

You will see from this that I was on a deficit diet and cut calories by about 900 kcal.

I was always hungry and more importantly could lose no weight, indeed, when I did consume slightly more carbohydrates I put weight on. Basically my body was in starvation mode and ensured that my fat cells clawed everything it could from the food I consumed.

The following shows more or less my macronutrient consumption once I'd embarked on the Ketogenic diet

Carbohydrates 20 grams = 80 calories

Protein 100 grams = 400 calories

Fat 140 grams = 1260 calories

Total calories = 1740

Here you will see that I am still in deficit, but taking in more nutrients, and my carbohydrate intake is minuscule. Because the type of carbohydrates I consume is nutrient dense and low glycemic, it means they do not cause my insulin to spike to high or for too long, and very little fat is created and exported to my fat cells as a result of carbohydrate consumption. In the main the fat that enters my cells are a result of fat consumption which is about 73% of what I consume on a daily basis.

Energy

Because I've cut carbohydrate consumption, my body needs to get energy from somewhere, so it has turned to its' secondary source, which is fat, and the more I continue with the diet the more fat I'll burn. Do you now see how this diet targets fat?

Getting Started: The things You'll Need

Weighing Scales:

To get started I needed no prompting and because I was always on some form of diet, I'd already bought myself a set of electronic scales. I know, I know, some of you are loath to using scales when preparing food. But these are essential, well, at least when you start. After a while you may learn how much 20 grams of coconut oil or 50 grams of avocado looks like, but if you're serious about losing weight, just bite the bullet and ensure that you get yourself a set.

Supplements:

Right now for every gram of carbohydrate you consume, your body holds on to 3 grams of water. When you go on to the diet and because of its nature, you will lose water and fat quickly. So you're going to need the following supplements:

Multivitamins with a good B complex (One in the morning at breakfast)

Potassium (Three 99mg in the morning at breakfast and two at night)

Magnesium (One 300gm in the morning at breakfast and one at night)

Increase sodium (salt) intake by 3 grams (Preferably Himalayan Pink salt)

Increase water intake

I made the mistake of not completing my research before starting the diet and found myself feeling very tired by the end of the first week. This was because my electrolytes, you know, salts, potassium and magnesium were being flushed out of my body. So it is very important that you take these consistently. Even the quantities I've outlined may be a little low, as some advocates say that those on ketogenic diets should take at least 3000mg of potassium and 900mg of magnesium per day, and increase sodium intake by about 3000mg. After I increased my intake of these I felt fine.

Special Foods:

In the first weeks you may become constipated, this is because you may not be consuming sufficient fat/oil, or drinking enough water, not getting enough fibre or consuming too much protein.

Well let's start with fibre: On the diet you will be eating leafy green vegetables such as cabbage, lettuce, kale, spinach, broccoli etc. Which should provide some fibre, however, you may want to use ground Flax seeds as I do, or Chia and Hemp seeds. I would advise that you take a table spoon (5 grams) of one of these on a daily basis.

You may also want to take, as I did in my first few weeks, Digestive Enzymes, which will aid the digestion; these can be bought as a supplement from good health food stores. Sauerkraut (fermented cabbage) contains natural enzymes and also aids digestion. I consume a small amount of sauerkraut every day and have no digestion issues.

As I said earlier, you must increase your water intake and as for the fat/oil consumption, I'll cover the amounts you should intake shortly as this will vary from person to person.

Protein:

Protein consumption will also vary from person to person and should fall within the advised recommended daily intake of between 0.8 grams and 1.2 grams (depending on how active you are) per kilogram of lean body weight. And when I say lean body weight, I mean your weight with the fat removed. How can I calculate that? I hear you ask. Well that's quite straight forward; there are many web sites that will do the calculation for you. In many cases, all you'll be required to do is to enter your gender, age and a few measurements and the web site will do the rest.

The sites usually return your body fat as a percentage figure, so if my total weight is 87.5 kilos and the site returns my fat percentage as 19%, to get my lean body weight I would have to remove 19% from 87.5 kilos, the calculation being 19 ÷ 100 x 87.5 = 16.62 which is my fat percentage expressed in kilos. I then remove the fat weight from my total weight, 87.5 - 16.62 = 70.88 would be my lean body mass.

The amount of protein that I would require would be calculated like this: 0.8 x 70.88 = 56 grams per day, if I am inactive or, 1.2 x 70.88 =85 grams per day if I frequent the gym on a regular basis, or more if I'm very active. I.E. lifting heavy weights body building, do a very active job, or are a sports person. I personally consume a little more protein than is recommended as a daily intake, as I am active at the gym most days.

Your protein should also contain fat, so rather than chicken breast, choose chicken thigh. You really need to use those meat fats, but remember this is not "Atkins", so refrain from over consuming protein.

Now that I've shown you the calculations which you may find daunting; I can indeed tell you that there are many websites that will do all the calculations for you. As with the body fat calculators, all you'll need to do is answer a few questions, like your gender, age and weight etc. Obviously, these type of websites work in a general way, so may not be one hundred percent accurate, but they worked for me. So take fifteen minutes out of your day to ensure you get your future protein consumption right.

Fat:

Consuming fat in this diet is the key to losing fat, as it will provide fuel for your body, has a brain calming effect among other things, and will not spike your blood sugar level, so you'll feel fuller for longer.

I started off by buying an oils high in Medium-chain Triglycerides (MCT) which means, and not wanting to bore you with a biology lesson, is readily absorbed and metabolised in the body. I used a mixture of an raw coconut oil, odorless coconut oil , Olive Oil, Butter/Dairy, pure 100% MCT oil and the oils from the meat and fish that I consumed. As well as using these, I ate avocados and nuts on a daily basis. My fat intake was and is still between 72% and 80% of my total calorie intake. For the diet to work, yours must be too.

It is important to note that you must not consume vegetable based fats/oils, as they are not as easy to digest and will make you fat. Also, you should not fry with the permitted oils/fats as you will change their composition. You can warm them, I.E. Use them in scrambled eggs, salad dressings, just pouring them over food or consuming them by the spoonful.

In the main, I consumed more raw and odorless coconut oils than anything else as I found them easy to use. I used the pure MCT oil as salad dressings and the butter in omelets, low heat stir-frys etc.

Carbohydrates:

For the first six weeks I kept my carbohydrate consumption to around 20 grams per day. Why? I'll explain why when I talk about getting your body into Ketosis.

Calorie Counting Websites and Apps:

Whilst on this diet you're going to have to count calories, and again I know many of you won't want to do this, however, as I said earlier, if you're serious about losing weight you'll find a way.

I calorie count because I know consuming a deficit will produce faster results and it has. I based my deficit on the recommended daily calorie intake for an average man of 2500 calories and when for a deep deficit of 30%, meaning that my daily intake would be in the region of 1750 calories per day. And as I pointed out earlier this meant I'd actually increased my macronutrient consumption.

It's up to you to choose a deficit, however, you don't have to, as the good thing about this diet is, even if you consumed the daily recommended amount, 2500 calories for a man and 2000 calories for woman, you would still lose fat as your body would be using it as its' primary source of energy.

There is help out there on the web: There are many sites which you can sign up to that will count calories for you. I've signed up to one where all you have to do is input the food you have consumed and it will give the calorific content, the fat, carbohydrate, protein and fibre content. Even foods from major stores can be found on their data bases, which makes things much easier. This way I have been able to plan my meals, and once planned, I'm able to weigh it out, either to eat that day or take to work with me the following day. Some of the best websites also provide APPs for smart phones and tablets, enabling you to input what you consume when you're on the go.

So to recap: You'll need to:

Take multivitamins

Take Potassium

Take Magnesium

Increase sodium (salt) intake

Increase water intake

Eat fibre and/or digestive enzymes

Work out how much protein you'll require and only increase if you become active

Get the right types of fats

Work out your body fat and sign up to a websites that will count calories

Seems like a lot of things to do, doesn't it? But just think of the results you'll gain....

Chapter 3: Getting Your Body into Ketosis, and Carbohydrate Types

Getting your body into ketosis means getting your liver to start producing "Ketone Bodies", the substance that will feed your brain while your body fat, the fat you consume and a portion of the ketone bodies sustains you.

It can be difficult to achieve this, but if you follow the steps I've laid out, most of you will. It took me two or three weeks to get my body into Ketosis, as even with the research that I had undertaken my diet was still a bit hit or miss. I was still consuming too many carbohydrates.

Depending on what is currently happening within your body hormonally, in some extreme cases it could take as long as three months to get into Ketosis, so be patient, because like me you've probably been overweight for years, so waiting another three months to become fat adapted will be a drop in the ocean. But you will still lose some weight.

So, plan your meals and consume the correct macronutrients: Your daily carbohydrate intake needs to be no more than 20 grams per day. For example 100 grams of Savoy cabbage may only contain 6.10 grams of carbohydrates and 50 grams of sauerkraut 2.1 grams. The websites I talked about in the last chapter will help you decide what to eat, but when to eat is a different matter. You should consume 70% of your carbohydrates for breakfast, mid morning snack and lunch, rather than leaving their consumption till the end of the day.

Your protein consumption should be spread evenly throughout the day which will allow for efficient metabolic absorption, and your fat consumption, as with the carbohydrates, 70% for breakfast, mid morning snack and lunch.

How will I know when I am in Ketosis I suppose will be your next question. Well there are bodily indicators that will let you know. Because you won't be holding water, your breath will begin to smell, which is commonly known as Keto Breath. NO! Not in a really horrible way, but you should notice it, just drink more water. Also your urine will begin to smell sweet as your body begins to dump the ketone bodies that it does not use.

There is a more scientific way to test to see if your body is producing ketones, and that is by using Keto Strips. There are many products on the market, but essentially this is a product that's used to test for the presence of ketones in the body: You urinate on them, and they change colour if ketones are present. If they do change colour, you know that you are in ketosis, but begin using these after two weeks of being on the diet.

Remember if you don't get into ketosis within two to three weeks, it's probable that you're still consuming to many carbohydrates; 20 grams per day is all you need to begin with. The types of carbohydrates that you consume may also be the issue; remember only consume low glycemic, green leafy vegetables. I'll list what I consumed a bit later. Or it may be that you're consuming too much protein, as eating too much protein causes your body to produce glucose, which raises your blood sugar levels, which is something you must avoid.

Keto Flu

Unfortunately some of you may get something which is called Keto Flu: This is not real flu, but it can be as draining. What's happening, is your body is going through sugar /glucose withdrawal, leaving you feeling tired and possibly with headaches. Just continue to drink plenty of water, take the Potassium, Magnesium and Increase sodium (salt) intake. This will help, it certainly did with me. You may get itchy skin or a rash, this will be because excess sugar loving parasites that live inside your body will begin to die, however this will pass.

OK, now that I've imparted my knowledge of this diet onto you, I do advise that you do a little research of your own. You may want to consult your physician, who will probably tell you that embarking on this diet is folly, and you should stick to a balanced diet. You know the diet that made you fat in the first place. But it is entirely your choice, as it was for me.

Most importantly, this diet is not right for everyone, and I would advise that type 1 diabetics do not do it. Vegetarians and Vegans will have to look closely at their protein and carbohydrate balance. And people that are prone to kidney stones or have rare metabolic conditions, gallbladder disease, pancreatic issues, are naturally thin, or have had bariatric surgery (gastric bypass), will have to think hard before embarking on this diet.

Carbohydrate Types

Foods to avoid: Includes all starchy food such as Potatoes, Rice, Pasta, Bread, processed foods containing added sugars, wheat and corn flours, vegetable based oils, and yes fruit. Fruits contain lots of sugars and shouldn't be consumed with in the first three weeks, or until you become fat adapted. After this time, you may have small portions of fruit high in antioxidants, such as Blueberries, Strawberries, Blackberries and Raspberries, and after five weeks or a few weeks after becoming fat adapted, one quarter of an apple or orange per day.

The carbohydrates listed below are what you can eat, however, no more than 20 grams of carbohydrate content per day. Remember 100 grams of savoy cabbage only contains 6.10 grams of carbohydrate and 50 grams of avocado contains 4.6 grams.

List of Some Carbohydrates That Are Low Glysimic

Eat Frequently:

Endive, Bok Choy, Broccoli Raab, Celery, Arugula,
Asparagus, Chard, Chayote, Eggplant, Hearts of Palm,
Lettuce, Radishes, Spinach, Green Cabbage, Green & Savoy,
Cauliflower, Cucumber, Daikon, Kohlrabi, Mushrooms,
Button, Pumpkin Puree, Rhubarb, Summer Squash, Zucchini
Avocado, Fennel
Green Beans, Mushrooms, Crimini & Oyster, Okra,
Radicchio, Tomatoes

Less Frequently:
Bell Peppers, Mushrooms, Enoki Turnips Artichoke
Brussels Sprouts, Red Cabbage, Snow Peas, Sugar Snap Peas,
Pumpkin, Turnip

Even less Frequently:
Carrots, Celeriac, Edamame , Winter Squash, Onion, Kale,
Jicama

What is on the menu:

Mustard Greens

Parsley (Chopped)

Spinach (Raw)

Bok Choi

Endive

Lettuce (Iceberg)

Lettuce (Romaine)

Sprouts Alfalfa

Lettuce (Boston Bibb)

Turnip Greens (Boiled)

Radicchio

Broccoli florets

Cauliflower (Steamed)

Garlic (Fresh)

Radishes

Cucumber (Raw)

Nopales (Grilled)

Pepper (Jalepeno)

Cabbage (Green Raw)

Mushroom (Shitake Cooked)

Squash (Summer)

Cabbage (Red Raw)

Cauliflower (Raw)

Mushroom (Button)

Squash (Zuchinni Steamed)

Asparagus (Steamed)

Cabbage (Green Steamed)

Fennel fresh

Cabbage (Savoy Steamed)

Artichoke (Hearts)

Broccoli Rabe

Collard Greens

Bean Sprouts

Eggplant (Broiled)

Kale steamed

Sauerkraut

Spinach (Steamed)

Tomato (Plum)

Turnips (Boiled)

Scallions

Jicama (Raw)

Tomato (Tomatillo)

Green Beans steamed

Yellow Wax Beans

Celery (Raw)

Peas (Snow)

Pepper (Green Bell)

Pepper (Red Bell)

Okra (Steamed)

Mushroom (Portabello)

Pumpkin (Canned)

Pumpkin (Boiled)

Brussel Sprouts (Steamed)

Okra (Fried)

Onion (Chopped)

Carrot (Steamed)

Rutabaga

Tomato (Cherry)

Carrot (Raw)

Peas (Regular)

Broccolini

Artichoke (Whole)

Waterchestnuts

Squash (Spaghetti)

Squash (Butternut Baked)

Squash (Acorn Baked)

Carbohydrate cycling whilst in Ketosis (Also known as Carb Cycling, Back Loading or Re-feeding)

Once in ketosis, some people do what is called carb cycling. This is when in the week they consume a ketogenic diet, however at the weekend or on one day of the week they carb up, by eating things like potato, rice, pasta and bread. There are differing views on this practice, where advocates of carb cycling say that, this actually helps them to burn fat, as consuming carbohydrates once a week effects the hormones that are related to the metabolism and fat loss. They believe that this practice is good for those whose weight has reached a plateau.

Kitogenic purists on the other hand would advise not to carb cycle, as this may lead to eating disorders brought on by the rising of other hormones. Their belief is that if you eat regularly throughout the day, your hormones will be fine. I went along with the keto purists and have not carb cycled. I am still losing fat and my metabolism is fine.

Alcohol:

Beer, Ales, ciders, sweet wines and shots are off the menu, they contain too much sugar and will prevent you getting into ketosis, and will kick you out of the state once you have reached it.

I only consumed alcohol once I'd been in ketosis for four weeks and then the only drinks I could drink were low no sugar spirits like vodka, dark rum, gin with no sugar mixers. And only the driest of wines will do, like sparkling white wine (brut) and reds such as Cabernet Sauvignon, Merlot and Cabernet Franc.

Chapter 4: Motivation and Suggested Daily Intake

To get me into ketosis, I consumed the same things throughout the day for three weeks. A bit boring I know, but I was focused, which is something you'll need to be.

Perhaps you've got at dress you have to fit into in a couple of months time, or suit trousers that have got too tight. No matter what it is, set a goal: I bought a pair of trousers two sizes too small, and two T-shirts one size too small. The goal was to fit into them within six months. Two and half months later, and my waste is three sizes smaller, and my T-Shirts size, two sizes smaller, what a waste of money! Well in a good way.

You may want to take a full body selfie from week to week to chart your progress, or get a group of friends to join you. As I said, we are all different and some of you may get into ketosis sooner than others and you never know, you may be needed to encourage someone, or may need encouragement yourself.

MOTIVATE YOURSELF! Just imagine and keep reminding yourself of size you want to be and it will happen.

Listed on the following pages are the meals I consumed that would take me into ketosis (being fat adapted) within three weeks. I haven't included a calorie count, as I want you to sign up to a site that count calories as I did and let them count the calories for you.

Breakfast	Lunch	Dinner	Snacks
Two medium eggs boiled, Coconut oil 20g, Butter 10g, Sauerkraut 25g, Cheddar Cheese 15g, Avocado 50g	Chicken Thighs 100g, Pork tender loin 50g, Green cabbage 50g, coconut oil 20g, butter 10g	Pork tender loin 80g, Cauliflower 50g, coconut oil 20g, butter 10g, Avocado 25g	Walnuts 28g, double cream 30g, Milled flax seeds 5g , Peanut butter 5g

Or

Breakfast	Lunch	Dinner	Snacks
Two medium eggs boiled, Coconut oil 20g, Butter 10g, Sauerkraut 25g, Back bacon 2 rashers, Avocado 50g	Corned beef 100g, Bok choi 100g, coconut oil 20g, butter 10g,	Chicken thigh 100g, Cauliflower 50g, Spinach 50g, Coconut oil 20g	Walnuts 28g, Milled flax seeds 5g, Peanut butter 5g

Add bacon, high meat / fat content sausages or spring greens, any combination, it's all good, really! And if you feel hungry then eat, things like a tea spoon full of peanut butter, or Tahini (sesame butter), or coconut manna; these will kill your cravings. Here are a few more daily meal ideas.

Breakfast	Lunch	Dinner	Snacks
Two medium eggs boiled, Coconut oil 20g, Butter 10g, Sauerkraut 25g, Back bacon 2 rashers, Avocado 50g	Corned beef 100g, Bok choi 100g, Artichoke 50g, coconut oil 20g, butter 10g,	Chicken thigh 100g, Boiled carrots 50g, Spinach 50g, MCT OIL 20g	Walnuts 28g, Milled flax seeds 5g, Peanut butter 5g

Breakfast	Lunch	Dinner	Snacks
2 high meat content sausages, Coconut oil 20g, MCT 10g, Sauerkraut 25g, Cheddar cheese 30g Avocado 50g	Rump steak 100g, Green cabbage 50g, boiled Carrots 30g, Coconut oil 20g, butter 10g	Grilled Salmon 100g, Cauliflower 50g, Spinach 50g, MCT OIL 20g	Walnuts 28g, Milled flax seeds 5g, Coconut Manna 15g

Breakfast	Lunch	Dinner	Snacks
2 high meat content sausages, Coconut oil 20g, MCT 10g, Sauerkraut 25g, Cheddar cheese 30g Avocado 50g	Sauerkraut 25g, Coconut oil 20g, Sautéed kidneys 80g, Sautéed pork liver 80g, Butter 20g	Chicken thigh 100g, Lettuce 50g, Sliced Tomato 80g, MCT OIL 20g	Walnuts 28g, Milled flax seeds 5g, Peanut butter 15g

There's a world of resource for meals, recipes and types of foods on the web; do your research.

Chapter 5: How Long Do You Stay In Ketosis

As mentioned earlier, this is a life style change that you'll have adopted, and it'll be up to you for how long you want to stay fat adapted.

I've been in Ketosis for several months and have had no side effects, indeed, I feel great. I'm full of energy, my blood pressure and cholesterol are good and my body hasn't looked this good in: I don't know; too many years to count.

After I'd lost 21 pounds, I went on and lost 5 more, which all in all took three months. I am now as lean as I want to be and my diet is now just maintenance.

After two months I raised my carbohydrate intake to 30 grams per day, and then at the three month mark, to 50 grams per day. My fat intake is still approximately 72% to 80% of my daily intake, and my protein consumption remains the same. My calorie count varies between 1900 kcal and 2300 kcal depending on how hungry I feel, and my weight is stable.

This diet works for me, and I am pretty sure it can work for you too. I believe the science to be sound, but check it out for yourself.

If you're fed up of being called "big guy", "big man", or someone who you haven't seen in a long time commenting on your weight without saying that you're fat: You know the usual comments. "Oh! You look well", or "Have you lost weight?" Become fat adapted. Get your body into ketosis and lose weight.

Oh! There are just a couple other things I'd like to comment on:

The first being exercise.

Even if you're not like me, a 'gym rat', and don't like to, or believe that you do not have enough time to do some sort of activity that raises your heart rate. I strongly advise that you begin to take some form of exercise. Even if you get out and walk for twenty minutes every day, that'll be better than just doing nothing. Tend your garden, take up Yoga or Pilates, just do something, because when the fat begins to fall away you may end up with unsightly sagging skin. So do some exercise to keep yourself toned.

The second thing is rest.

You must try to relax and take rest periods where necessary. It is also important that you get a good night's sleep, as when you sleep growth hormones are produced and they'll help with the fat burn. The optimum time where you'll get the most benefit from these hormones is between 10pm and 2am, so try to relax and get your head down early.

If you require any help or advice, contact me on the following email address.

lose-weight@hotmail.com

Anyway that's it from me, and I hope this helps.

ABOUT THE AUTHOR

Daniel McKenzie though not a nutritionist has a passion for food, indeed, he almost paid for some overindulgences with his life a few years ago. It was while convalescing he would decide to write his first novel.

He has since lost 7 stones in weight, and feels that there are many people like him, whose bodies cannot handle the modern carbohydrates and sugar packed foods that we consume on a daily basis. He reiterates that he is no authority on nutrition, but as with his first novel, "A Thai Bride" published in 2012, here he has written about what he believes, and knows within his heart will change the lives of many people for the better.

Educated to college standard, Daniel had spent 12 years catering industry, 30 years in the music / media industry before turning his hand to writing, and is now looking at sports training and nutrition to be at the forefront to the next chapter of his life.

Printed in Great Britain
by Amazon.co.uk, Ltd.,
Marston Gate.